How To Naturally Reverse Diabetes:

Can You Cure Diabetes Naturally?

Copyright 2013

Table of Contents

Common Sense Medical Disclaimer   4

Tons of Information on the Diabetic Diet
and Other Helpful Resources   5

Gestational Diabetes Diet and
Gestational Diabetes Symptoms   13

Juvenile Diabetes Symptoms:
Jenn's Story and What to Watch For   19

Fenugreek and Type Two Diabetes   21

Omega-3 and the Diabetic Diet Resources   24

Gymnema and Diabetes:
Our Past and The Introduction of Gymnema   27

Gymnema Will Make You Eat Less Sugar and
Lose Weight! Is that True About Gymnema? Read on!   32

Health Benefits From Cinnamon   34

The Diabetic Diet and A1C levels?   38

How can Processed Food Alter
the Diabetic Diet?   40

Glycine Propionyl L-Carnitine:
Part Amino Acid Part Fat Eater!   42

Diabetic Diet Resources During
the Summertime   44

Water Is Your New Diabetic Diet
Resources Best Friend!   46

WHY is Alkaline Water Important?   48

Alkaline Water : Do It Yourself Style!   50

Fast Diabetic Diet Resources   52

Naturally Lower Blood Sugar Levels
With Food?   54

Diabetic Blunders and Myths To Avoid!   56

Some More Myths for You!   58

Is There A Diabetic Exercise?   62

An Important Task – Weight Management   65

Focus on This Weight Management Tip For Success!   67

Weight Management – You have to Believe In It!   70

You Made It This Far!   73

Common Sense Medical Disclaimer

I am NOT a doctor, I do not play one, and I will not pretend to be one. Diabetes is a serious condition that will kill you if not treated properly. Listening to the advice of, and adhering to the advice of, your primary endocrinologist or doctor overseeing the care of your diabetes should be of paramount information.

I will not and cannot diagnose, treat, prevent, or cure your condition. All I can do is provide the information I have learned through years of non-specialized study (I have a degree, just not in medicine or any related field).

If there's anything you find of interest in here, and that is the whole point, you really must bring it to your doctor's attention before trying anything out. That's not just with what you will learn in this book, but anything you may attempt in life.

Tons of Information on the Diabetic Diet and Other Helpful Resources

Why would you consider the diabetic diet resources in this book as a safe haven? To find out simply read on! Drowning in the middle of the Atlantic Ocean sounds scary, does a diagnosis of diabetes sound equally terrifying? It should, with all the information and changes required regarding diet and lifestyle, there stands a fair chance this condition could take your life or at a minimum, greatly diminish your quality of life That is of course if you allow it to. In life, knowledge is power and when it comes to diabetes that fact is no different.

Through the years, there have been tremendous gains in the realm of diabetic information. We know a lot more about alternative treatments coupled with long-standing treatments and how they can work well together. I've learned the worst thing you can have with diabetes is fear, the tips and ideas in this book are meant to help alleviate some of those fears through gained knowledge.

I will say upfront that I am not a doctor or any type of endo-specialist. I will say however that I am a prolific reader and I love studying numerous health topics, especially medical conditions. What led me to reading into what we know and what we can do about diabetes is the effect it had on a few family members as well as close friends. I saw their downs, and I saw their remarkable high's when they got serious about their health and took it into their own hands.

If I'm Not A Doctor, Why Listen To Me?

That's a great question that I would love to answer, it comes from work experience and a passion for change! I began really looking into diabetes as it was my job, literally. I was employed for a few years by a nutritional supplement chain, and we had a very large amount of customers who were living with diabetes. It was my job to give them useful and actionable information.

I didn't just want to give information, I wanted to know inside and out the why and how to answers. Anyone can give an answer, I wanted to give more. Many of the customers dealing with diabetes sought me out specifically to answer their diabetic related questions. I was a trusted source of information, and that wasn't something I took lightly!

It wasn't only my job, I was facing being diagnosed with diabetes myself! I refused to let such a devastating condition take me, so I fought back.

When working at a Vitamin World I saw so many nervous customers come in that were on the verge or having just been diagnosed with Type II Diabetes, I could pick them out before they would tell me exactly what they were looking for.

Just like with treating diabetes, I always had a specific starting point. I always wanted to know what they knew about their blood sugar patterns. Asking them how they controlled their blood sugar was the easiest way for me to see what they were doing obviously.

Spending a ton of money on blood sugar controlling herbs was not always needed, especially when some can interfere with a medicine they could have been taking! As I increased my research on the topic, it was always evident that minerals and herbs do work, very well for that matter, however are most powerful when used along with a diabetic diet and under the direct supervision after receiving approval from a doctor. I began really looking into diabetic diet resources and the changes were not difficult or hard to manage at all if done incrementally and with a strategic plan of sorts (not just trying something for a week for example).

After I was Scared Straight I "Met" the Diabetic Diet

I read constantly on the topic of the diabetic diet, read into various diabetic diet tips, and was told at a routine doctor's visit I was on the verge of diabetes type two. That was not going to happen nor was I going to consider medicine, especially when I read how manageable and reversible type two diabetes is. I have personally been against medicine most of my life, it's just not something I was interested in doing (a pill a day for life sounds too prisoner-esque personally). Again, that is my personal decision based on the information I took in.

Numerous diabetic diet resources mentioned in this book such as willpower as well as portion control are fundamental and extremely important aspects of this diet and the principals in this book. Are you wondering "why will power" would be something of paramount importance when trying to better your diabetic treatment, including the "diabetic diet"? Let's take a peak, and then you should firmly understand why willpower is extremely important when discussing diabetes.

Let The Basic Understandings Proceed

This is going to be one of the longer chapters in this book, and it's going to briefly touch on a bunch of different topics. We'll cover many of them more indepthly, however this chapter is going to be sort of like the pre-algebra class you took in high school before studying full blown algebra. Let's get started by briefly "studying" how our food's history has adapted, negatively, to our changing views and lifestyle.

Our last few generations in America have began using food as a reward and a reason to celebrate instead of its true purpose, which is to survive. It should become a little more obvious why the diabetic diet resources I read mentioned will power as a focal point. Portion control should be a little more obvious, especially due to the fact that type two diabetes is many times the result of a poorly managed diet. Not just a poorly constructed and consumed diet but also the correlation between that as well a lack of willpower. We'll look into willpower later, but for now we're going to cover diet.

So What Should We Look Into Eating?

Without consuming the proper foods, you could be wasting your time with the diabetic diet. The diet is no different from the one and one equals two mathematically equation. When you begin the diet, portion control added with the proper food choices equals the diabetic diet equation. And we'll also be going against "common knowledge" which state that carbohydrates need to be avoided.

We're not just going to be eating carbs, we're going to eat more of them than protein! In fact, you'll want to make sure half of your plate consists of carbohydrates. We're not talking bread and pasta, the cars you're going to want to eat are called complex carbohydrates, these are mainly going to be in the form of vegetables.

The vegetables (complex carbohydrate containing foods) you want to have as a majority on your plate are the non-starchy types such as cauliflower and broccoli. These aren't the only veggies you'll be consuming but I've found that they contain a whole bunch of really good for you phytonutrients and vitamins! Plus they're fibrous, and what I consider to be super veggies.

I mentioned that broccoli and cauliflower aren't the only veggies you'll be consuming for your complex carbs. A few other vegetables you'll want to add are carrots, eggplant, and different types of peppers.

Seeing half of our plate is now full, you want to mentally cut the remaining portion in half, creating two quarters. One of the quarters will have a serving of simple carbohydrates or starchy foods such as rice or cooked beans. The remaining portion will be a protein such as lean beef, chicken or turkey, or maybe fish if you enjoy it and can get past the smell. Actually, as we'll see later in this book, fish may not bad a bad idea at all after we learn what omega-3 can do for you!

Can We Touch a Little More On Carbohydrates Please?

Especially with the Atkin's Diet, we've been told from all angles to steer clear of carbs, but if we did we'd be taking a ton of nutritional supplements to get the raw health power the right ones provide. Even the "wrong" or starchy carbohydrates are not horrible in moderation (unless they are extremely processed and provide zero nutritional benefits).

Carbohydrates come in two forms, as mentioned earlier. The biggest difference between simple and complex carbohydrates is how our bodies break them down. One of the carbohydrates takes very little time to raise blood sugar, this is the simple form of carbohydrates. These are the carbohydrates a diabetic will take to spike their blood sugar after it drops.

Complex carbohydrates take longer to be broken down by the body and will not raise blood sugar as fast. These carbohydrates can be taken in conjunction with a simple carbohydrate to stabilize the blood sugar once it has risen, this would be a hummus or peanut butter normally.

How's YOUR Mineral Intake Looking?

Diabetics hold the notorious attribute of being deficient in minerals including chromium. This is especially true for those with type two diabetes, which is why mineral supplements are a popular dietary additive after research. In fact, you may want to ask your doctor about chromium as well as magnesium, two minerals I'm going to cover.... now. Actually, I'm going to give you some "pre-algebra" into why you want to have minerals in your diet first, then I will discuss the I promise.

Minerals are equally important to biochemical reactions in your body as vitamins are and greatly deal with controlling blood sugar. Minerals are also known to decrease your insulin resistance, which is a common diabetic issue. In fact, many of the foods mentioned in the diabetic diet are mineral rich aside from providing vitamin and phytonutrient properties to your food's true goodness.

Chromium is by far the most popular supplement I saw being purchased for blood sugar control, and when researching diabetic diet resources, this was normally the first one mentioned. Why does chromium have such a popular hold in the world of the diabetic diet and natural diabetes supplements? I will say first that all individuals need it as it does a wonderful job of breaking down fats and carbohydrates during metabolization.

Another important and often times deficient in diabetics, mineral is magnesium. Magnesium is an important factor in over 300 separate biochemical functions and processes in the body including the control of blood sugar levels.

Aside from helping to stabilize blood sugar levels, magnesium also helps to lower glucose levels during fasting, which is an action that is not necessarily safe for diabetics to do outside of a doctor's care.

Although not as well known for their health related properties, non-mineral supplements can also help regulate blood sugars and can be included in the diabetic diet!

Cinnamon, although not a mineral, is one of these supplements and food choices, which is slowly becoming accepted as a blood sugar controlling tool. In fact, cinnamon is becoming encouraged as a part of the diabetic diet by more and more health professionals.

The reason behind this is positive studies show the effect of cinnamon and the safety as well as availability of it. Cinnamon has not been shown to counteract with oral diabetic medicines and in fact helps them regulate blood sugar more efficiently.

Cinnamon isn't the only non-veggie/protein/mineral that is thought to be awesome for diabetes. There are other herbs and natural remedies that serve many purposes as well as potentially being beneficial to diabetes such as gymnema, fenugreek, and ginseng.

Gymnema has been used for a variety of medical treatments around the country of India as well as portions of Africa for thousands of years. Gymnema is by far the most popular plant form herb that is used to treat diabetes as it makes the body's cells more receptive to insulin and decreases resistance.

Ginseng is normally thought of as only an herb that promotes energy, not true. Among the variety of uses ginseng has, specifically North American ginseng, is its ability to better control blood sugars. I do not condone dropping or starting anything without first consulting your endocrinologist!

The diabetic diet is popular and has shown numerous times it will help reverse the effects of type two diabetes and the prediabetic conditions. There really is no reason your doctor or a nutritionist will discourage you from taking on the diabetic diet.

Actually there is one and this should be a stark reminder why you pay them to help you. We're not robots and your unique situation is going to be different than mine. Aside from embarking on the diabetic diet, ask your doctor how they feel about the inclusion of herbal supplements in your new regiment! Don't be discouraged by their answers, herbs and such are only really getting looked into on the medical level now, although they have been used in the same sense for millenniums (literally). Your doctor may just not know about them yet.

Gestational Diabetes Diet and Gestational Diabetes Symptoms

This one is geared toward, but not only, the ladies unless the daddy to-be's are afraid of developing gestational diabetes symptoms themselves but you can follow the gestational diabetes diet with mommy! Kidding aside, us guys cannot get gestational diabetes. When speaking about managing the "Big D", or as most refer to as diabetes, you almost never hear about a gestational diabetes diet.

A gestational diabetes diet could be intricately important in ensuring that the diabetes only stays the length of the pregnancy! Gestational diabetes symptoms can appear to stay after you bring in your bundle of joy, however the symptoms can often be linked to diabetes type 2. If you stick to the gestational diabetes diet, this issue should avoid you! This concept is especially true if personal care after the baby has come leads to poor dietary habits. It is extremely possible to play it smart and get your former physique and health back by deeply considering the gestational diabetes diet.

Will the Gestational Diabetes Diet lower your Risk of Gestational Diabetes? Actually, what raises the risk first!

Actually before we jump into the gestational diabetes diet let's take a quick peek at what raises your risk of developing gestational diabetes symptoms and the condition itself. If you are around 20% higher than your normal body weight, your risks are highly elevated. You always hear that it is important to maintain a healthy body weight. Another factor toward your risk is being of ethnic persuasion such as Native American, Black, Asian, etc, meaning you should really consider some form of a gestational diabetes diet.

Another common sign you are on the verge or are showing gestational diabetes symptoms is done at the doctors office by you having blood in your urine. The gestational diabetes diet could reduce these risk factors and effects over time. Again, these have worked in some people but you still need to do your own homework.

Gestational diabetes symptoms are normally rare. Actually only about 4%, at the time of this writing, of expectant mothers are diagnosed with gestational diabetes regardless, the risk is there. Although the rates are only 4%, this is not something with which you would want to play roulette as gestational diabetes symptoms can and normally do affect baby as well.

Following a gestational diabetes diet or something similar can reduce the risks associated with gestational diabetes. I'll mention it again, the gestational diabetes diet is not a complex endeavour! Actually, the gestational diabetes diet was one of the easier health changes I undertook (I am a guy, however I was cooking for a diabetic)! I am not saying it is super easy to stick to the gestational diabetes diet immediately, however it can happen with diligence.

Diagnosis of this condition is tough to come by. Normally gestational diabetes symptoms are hidden and do not usually show. The way gestational diabetes is normally found is by blood work. Some of the symptoms include extreme or regular thirst, hunger attacks, or you will show signs of hypoglycemia which could actually, if you think about it, be gestational diabetes symptoms. Here's a fast run down of hypoglycemia:

- Confusion
- Dizziness
- Feeling shaky or unsteady
- Headaches
- Sudden hunger
- Weakness

Remember, the gestational diabetes diet if managed and used properly should reduce your hypoglycemia risks! Actually, the gestational diabetes diet is pretty easy to follow and the gestational diabetes diet can be used after your baby comes!

Onto the gestational diabetes diet! You want to aim for small meals three times daily. You also want to plan in 2 or 3 smaller snacks around the same time each day. Skipping meals or snacks isn't the world's best idea as this messes up the gestational diabetes diet's regularity and could affect your sugar more than desired. Carbohydrates are going to be broken up into 40%-45% in the morning (the amount is based on the total calorie intake, ie you want to aim for carbs being 45ish% of your calorie intake).

The gestational diabetes diet also throws an odd number at you of between 15-30 grams of carbohydrates for a night time snack.

It may appear odd that there's an exact number but trust me, your body will be happy. If morning sickness is bugging you, keep a couple servings of crackers (wheat, come on we're getting healthy here!), cereal or pretzels which are dry foods and should make your baby a little happier. On the gestational diabetes diet you get to eat those snacks before getting out of bed, which is why you want a couple of servings near the bed stand. Another benefit of the gestational diabetes diet, you are allowed to snack (if you are feeling ill of course)

The gestational diabetes diet shares some commonalities with other diets. Fats are needed, however not in excess and the gestational diabetic diet is no different! In fact here are two percents for you, 10% of your total should be the only amount of saturated fats you consume, because they are bad for you! If anything, aim for a much lower number – if any. 40% or less of your caloric intake when on the gestational diabetic diet should be fats, and if at all possible should be along the omega line (omega 3).

Vegetables are going to become your friend if they are not already. In fact you may be wise to team them up with fiber seeing you should be aiming for around 35-40 grams of fiber daily (I bought a ton of Kashi cereals, 3 birds with one stone! Ok, only 2 stones). Seasonings will vary by taste and what baby likes but that's perfectly fine and you can use herbs (especially those with health benefits) to spruce up your meals.

Monitor your sodium intake as well seeing that gestational diabetes symptoms, especially hypoglycemia, do not need to be complicated by high blood pressure. Looking like the gestational diabetes diet can be used for a while yet? As I researched, the gestational diabetes diet appeared to be beneficial for most people!

If you show gestational diabetes symptoms regardless if you are following a gestational diabetes diet, you need to contact a medical professional immediately. What I learned with my ex-girlfriend is that regardless if you are on a gestational diabetes diet or if you have type one diabetes, which my ex-girlfriend does, your sugars will fluctuate. You should keep a note of your entire gestational diabetes diet consumption as well as your blood sugars! This is extremely important, as your baby will be affected by high and low blood sugar levels. Blood sugar levels will probably be off in the beginning and we were told this is to be expected as your body is going to go through major, natural, changes.

The gestational diabetes diet should help with these issues. Another occurrence that could happen is that they want you to stay in the hospital for a few days, this is extremely normal seeing that even if you are on a gestational diabetes diet your pregnancy will be considered higher risk. Again, this is very normal and helps your medical professionals see a small scope of how your body operates. My ex-girlfriend hates the hospital, but it was for the baby! With gestational diabetes the little bundle of joy needs to come first and you really need to consider mentioning the gestational diabetes diet with your doctor! The doctor I spoke with said she mentions the gestational diabetes diet to many of her patients, although she has a different name for it.

A great tip I'll follow (well, my ex-girlfriend) is to inform the doctor we'll be trying to have a baby. Actually, when we found out she was pregnant was the first time I had heard of the gestational diabetic diet. Actually, we were referred to a nutritionalist on the premise that after the baby came my ex-girlfriend would have access to some pretty awesome gestational diabetic diet resources. Actually, the best gestational diabetic diet or diabetic diet resource I will give you is to keep in touch with your doctor! I am not a doctor, nor am I pretending to be, I am just giving you all the gestational diabetes diet and gestational diabetes symptoms I have learned.

My son is 9 months old, and we still stick to the gestational diabetes diet. I will never have a child of my own as it is not physically possible (I am a man) however I am starting to see health effects by staying on the gestational diabetes diet! Actually, my fat levels since getting on the gestational diabetes diet have improved dramatically.

Consider the gestational diabetes diet for your life! Actually, if you want a nice diabetic diet resource consider the gestational diabetes diet for the following reasons; the gestational diabetes diet is very manageable, the gestational diabetes diet is easier than most to implement, the gestational diabetes diet can be full of vitamin rich foods!

On a closing note, the gestational diabetes diet is not a substitute for your prenatal vitamins! Do not start the gestational diabetes diet, nor stop taking your vitamins without your doctor's "ok". I have never heard a doctor say no to a gestational diabetes diet based meal plan!

Juvenile Diabetes Symptoms :
Jenn's Story and What to Watch For

Juvenile diabetes symptoms are something you need to be aware of as they are warning signs for an extremely serious condition! I have seen the ups and downs of diabetes in all its forms. The one that scares me the most, personally, is Type 1 symptoms, or juvenile diabetes symptoms are some of the worst. With juvenile diabetes symptoms it is extremely rare for a reversal, as the pancreas is pretty much just an object in your body that no longer serves a purpose. The symptoms for juvenile diabetes range, however there are some stark similarities in cases.

Juvenile Diabetes Symptoms and Jenn

What about the type 1 diabetes diet? Why wasn't it mentioned? We're going to stay away from that and read a small rundown of my ex-girlfriends experience with her juvenile diabetes symptoms, here we go!

"I had no idea what juvenile diabetes symptoms were, I know I felt really sick and very tired out of the blue. I had no energy, even at the start of the day. I couldn't concentrate in school either. I dropped a substantial amount of weight, and would feel sick to my stomach after only a sip or two of soda! I wasn't sure why I couldn't drink because I was always thirsty although I was hardly ever hungry, I never had an appetite! It's like I was a normal everyday kid getting into trouble around the house and out of the blue it's like something hit me. We found out the hard

way that I was diabetic. One day I just felt worse than I had lately and collapsed. I was rushed to the hospital and my sugar was around 1800, which is borderline diabetic coma levels!

I was laid up in the hospital for a little bit and the doctor told my mother all the warning signs I had were juvenile diabetes symptoms, even though I was a pre-teen. My life is not over yet in fact I live a very normal life. I just have to watch my sugar levels and make sure I am eating the right stuff. I still cheat once in awhile but have stable blood sugar levels on average and my A1C levels actually even dropped a little bit!"

It is of extreme importance if you think you are suffering from even just one of the mentioned juvenile diabetes symptoms to contact your doctor immediately. Don't be scared, nor surprised if he says he will meet you at the hospital! Do not ignore these basic juvenile diabetes symptoms. Are they all the juvenile diabetes symptoms? Absolutely not as everyone's juvenile diabetes symptoms will vary as we are not all robots.

Fenugreek and Type Two Diabetes

What is the deal with fenugreek and why is it becoming so popular fast, and why would they name it fenugreek? Let's uncover what fenugreek is and how fenugreek can help with ailments aside from diabetes!

When you think of a way to possibly beat the devastating condition diabetes you may imagine tons of tubes and dialysis like machinery correct? Some say that you can actually lower your blood sugar levels and blood glucose levels with a tiny, tiny seed known as fenugreek. Actually, fenugreek is gaining in popularity for its effects on people with, among other conditions, type two diabetes. Especially those who feel they can cure diabetes themselves or are trying to prevent diabetes after being diagnosed with pre-diabetes.

Fenugreek helps with more than diabetes!

Fenugreek seed is from the fenugreek plant which is normally grown and cultivated naturally around the Middle East as well as the Indian region and regions in Northern Africa such as Egypt. The plant must like the heat as those area's normally have very specific, and extremely warm, climates. Fenugreek has been used for numerous medical conditions as a treatment aside from diabetes including breast feeding – talk about total opposite ends of the health spectrum!

Onto the important stuff, how can a simple itty bitty seed such as fenugreek help reverse your diabetes when paired with traditional and other health practices? I can tell you that when I was pre-diabetic I was popping 500 mg of fenugreek twice a day. I would have taken the seed and used it as maybe a salad addition but finding fenugreek seed, not the extract, in the United States is near impossible unfortunately. When you can find it, it is normally relatively expensive however you may be able to get good deals at holistic healing centers.

This powerful herb is not something new, in facts it's much older than you may think. Fenugreek seed has actually been used for thousands of years in the area as a culinary treat as well as an area "cure all" for various ailments in it's regions of cultivation. On top of having medicinal attributes, fenugreek is also used in some tea's. Of course science has limited research on the topic of fenugreek as a blood sugar control agent as science is just starting to really study alternative health as additional treatments to traditional treatments.

What Makes Fenugreek So Effective Against Diabetes?

It's not the seed itself that has these awesome health benefits, like the old saying "it's what's inside that counts". One of these compounds hidden inside the nutrient rich fenugreek seed is 4-hydroxyisoleucine, which is a form of the amino acid isoleucine.

The American Diabetes Association has noted that their studies do in fact conclude that 4-hydroxyisoleucine contains the ability to act as an antidiabetic agent therefore reiterating the fact fenugreek does have the ability to fight off some diabetic effects and symptoms relating to blood sugar control.

So How Does It Work?

This blood sugar controlling amino acid is thought to stimulate insulin secretion, which is a good thing when you are battling high blood pressure as well. Some studies also conclude that taking too much of this can do some harm by increasing insulin resistance a little too much which will cause low blood sugar! Granted it's not high blood sugar, but you want a "happy medium" of sorts. Remember our diet? We want moderation, or a mid-level.

Another beauty inside these little fenugreek seeds are the amount of alkaloids such as trigonelline, carpaine, as well as gentianine. Never heard of these guys? I bet you have never heard of berberine either! Berberine is a natural plant-based alkaloid and is proven to be safe in the treatment of type two diabetes. In fact, HbA1c levels during a study went from $7.5 \pm 1.0\%$ to 6.6 ± 0.7, which over 3 months is a pretty substantial drop.

This particular alkaloid actually has shown to decrease triglyceride levels as well! Are you starting to see why I consider fenugreek to be as close to an all in one supplement as you can get? Fenugreek cooks (you do, but you know what I mean), it helps with blood sugar, type two diabetes, and so much more! If you can find the fenugreek seed you may even want to add fenugreek into your diabetic diet!

Omega-3 and the Diabetic Diet Resources

When you think of health encompassing resources beneficial to diabetes, what types of protein would you consider? I am not talking about Ensure or Syntha 6, I am talking as a chewable food and not a processed supplement. I'm hinting toward a really fishy and really good for you source of protein that has something really special in it (want to take a guess?).

Fish is one of my new found resources that I eat between 2 and 3 times weekly to keep diabetes from ever coming near me again (seriously, it gave me nightmares of lost limbs and everything). I say new found because for my first 28 and one half years of life, I was allergic to fish. This summer I found out it appears I outgrew my allergy and started eating fish a few times a week. The days I don't eat fish I'll take a couple 1200 milligram softgels. Omega 3 passes off some amazing heart health benefits! I make myself eat fish, the smell of it cooking drives me up the world.

Why Count Omega-3's As An Addition?

What can fish and omega-3 do for you as a diabetic and why would you want something on your diabetic diet resources sheet that causes stinky breath? There are a couple things actually, and I'll explain why your uptake of fish or omega 3 needs to be placed higher on your dietary priorities!

Omega-3 is a form of fatty acid that your body can actually use to help it function better! Also, when reading up on why my ex-

girlfriend, who is a type 1 diabetic, should add fish to her list of diabetic diet resources I found the answer. Consuming fish at least once a week is thought to help your body naturally control blood sugar!

We all know fish and omega-3 are brain foods, however what about one of the more important diabetes attack zones – your heart? Another reason fish instantly (upon me being able to consume it officially) hit my personal dietary arsenal is the amount of heart healthy positive attributes it has. Let's hit a few and slowly close the gap toward fish and omega-3 becoming one of your personal diabetic diet resources! Reducing strokes is always cool, right? This is accomplished by the omega-3 reducing inflammation in your body as well as blood clotting (those are two things you want to avoid having as part of your health's activities at all costs!)

Not Just The Oil

Fish isn't just full of omega 3, it is also has a very good amount of protein in it, and even better diet-wise is that it's lower on the caloric side! Muscle needs protein regardless if it is to fix a tear due to a strenuous exercise, don't forget that the organ you use all day is made of muscle (your heart).

As you already know, many of our diet resources contain strong sources of protein. Protein, as I mentioned does far more than simply fix muscles. It normally contains branched chain amino acids which are the building blocks of muscles. In the long run, and why I pick high protein foods for my diet plan, is that your body needs protein for everyday functions and not to be used as an energy source. That's another thing that makes fish containing good amounts of omega-3 one of my newest favorite diabetic diet resources is that it can be fatty which in turn adds a fuel source (as long as you're not a couch potato).

Have you ever heard the saying "that's food for thought"? That is another reason omega-3 should be considered one of your diabetic diet resources. Aside from the known heart health benefits, this diabetic diet mainstay (new for me, you should already be chowing down on it) is the brain feeding benefits it provides.

What's your brain made of? Matter and fat right? Wouldn't adding a good fat to a pile of fat make sense? Before you say no way, I said good fat so feel free to agree with me.

In the elderly, eating fish containing high levels of omega-3 is thought to reduce the risk of dementia as well as dementia-related cousins (a la Alzheimer's and other cognitive disorders and conditions). How about memory? I remember (no pun intended) that growing up as a child I was always told I was missing out because fish would help my memory and make me study less.

Gymnema and Diabetes:
Our Past and The Introduction of Gymnema

Gymnema sylvestre and diabetes are becoming a very popular "couple" over here in the United States of America. This is especially true lately as many are seeking other options to supplement their diabetes treatment. When looking around at US citizens from the outside inward, you will notice that we are a very odd or different culture than any other.

Different parts of this one country also have different moral and value sets than other parts of the country. The northern part of the country, specifically the North East for example, is strikingly different from the Southern states. New Englanders are fast paced and a stressful, of sorts, set of individuals. People in the South are far more laid back and take their time with things (and far more hospitable).

You may even notice we fancy, like a country, the kind of type two diabetes diet that would leave many scratching their heads and wondering "do they have any idea what they are doing to their bodies?" with proper reason. As a country, generally we have a severely horrible diet, so congratulations for trying to fix yours. Do not take that statement as an implication that we are purposely going out of our way and intentionally increasing our risk of diabetes. In fact, as a country we realize we are inducing type two diabetes when we could alter that path rapidly as well as extremely easily, but for some reason we just have not done that in the past.

Actually, the fact we are on the wrong diabetic diet has more or less been classified as "out of sight and out of mind", however we are cognoscente of it and that is a reason gymnema is starting to come up in conversation. We're creatures of habit and we enjoy the pleasures of food.

Lately, supplements like gymnema have been a popular course of action for inclusion in the diabetic diet as a nutritional supplement. One of the more popular supplements has been gymnema sylvestre. This course of action is pretty much needed as we fill our bodies regularly with unprocessed, trans fat filled junk food, greasy fast food, snacks, and many other food items that lack any nutritional benefits.

I'll say it again (because it really bothers me) that unfortunately,food is not seen as fuel, however more as a reward or activity. This is a leading factor toward why you could find us to be a peculiar set of people. This is where gymnema enters the equation and here is my argument as to how gymnema and diabetes are becoming a popular "couple" in regards to the bad or wrong diabetic diet, and how we can possibly reverse the effects of our current diet.

A Little Plant Called Gymnema Does What?

What makes gymnema stand out anyway, after all gymnema is only a plant right? You are correct that gymnema is a plant, however this plant is more of an "anti diabetic" Swiss army knife (remember fenugreek?)! Gymnema serves multiple uses and purposes. The most important property gymnema contains is the fact it has proven to stabilize blood sugar levels.

Aside from that, gymnema sylvestre goes far beyond diabetes in fact gymnema has been said to help with a variety of other

symptoms and conditions. Some other activities employed by gymnema are being antiviral, the lowering of cholesterol. Like fenugreek helping from diabetes to breastfeeding, here's how vast this plant's properties are – gymnema sylvestre has been noted as having the ability to reduce the effects of snake bites!

Gymnema sylvestre is carried by any decent natural supplement store such as Vitamin World or GNC. The supplement is normally sold in capsule, however I have seen (and used) it as a tincture or liquid substance (you'll definitely want to add it to something else!). Store's have carried it for a years now as a diabetic and blood sugar stabilizing agent, however in one of the countries of its origin, gymnema is seen as much more.

In India as well as isolated areas of Africa gymnema is said to (not proven in the US- yet) actually get rid of type two diabetes. In fact, when I first mentioned the diabetic type two diet jokingly, a person of Indian decent said it is not a new theory and they "use it in India all the time". Diabetes is actually a newer "mainstream" health concern in India, as obesity has not been entirely commonplace. This is because India has slowly been erasing its Third World status over the course of the last few decades. This should not be a problem as gymnema is literally right there waiting to help!

Gymnema is breaking through!

Although gymnema sylvestre has been gaining popularity lately, a couple groups have held this plant and extract as a treasure for over a century. Holistic healers as well as herbologists have given the plant praise for a very long time. The government and other authoritarian institutes are slower, with proper reason, to acknowledge the properties of natural items such as gymnema.

However, gymnema has caught the attention of a new and widely respected fan. That new fan is none other than the Harvard Medical School! This is going to be a massive popularity boost for this little wonder plant. Although alternative medicine and healing normally are a second thought due to the prevalence in our society of the pharmaceutical approach, gymnema's jump in fame could rapidly change that view.

Will alternative medicines and healing agents, such as gymnema sylvestre, overcome the powers of traditional pharmaceutical healing? No and for very good reason. Many natural remedies may have a known attribute or ability to aid in the healing of certain conditions; they widely have different effects on different people. For example, some people have a better result using gymnema as a weight loss aid when they are only trying to lower their blood sugar (but I'm sure they don't complain about the weight loss).

Gymnema is not the only oddball, another example of a, what I label them, "weird healer" is green tea where some have a thermogenic effect on them while others will find they are not losing weight however have a stronger immune system. I feel, and have zero scientific backing – just a wise hypothesis – this is because we are all individuals and are not mass-produced yet (kidding but you never know).

Why is gymnema seen as the "sugar destroyer"? Easy, another way of saying gymnema sylvestre is "gumar" which in Hindu, means literally "sugar destroyer". I don't know about you, however when I hear destroyer I instantly imagine a United States Naval ship or maybe an army. A simple, wimpy looking plant though? With its history and known attributes, I think those speaking Hindu labeled it very properly!

The type two diabetes diet is known to cause insulin to have an inability or a lack of effectiveness to process sugar, thus giving the body higher blood sugars. Gymnema is used to treat, as previously mentioned, diabetes by helping to make the cells in our body more receptive to insulin in turn lowering our blood sugar.

What about the destroyer, Gumar? That is simply another name for Gymnema. Although they do not say it directly, Harvard Medical School apparently believes the type two diabetes diet can be eased by allowing gumar (gymnema) to act as the" sugar destroyer".

So why should a case be made for gymnema sylvestre? For one, we covered the fact that for millenniums Indian and some African countries have used and acknowledged gymnema as having anti-diabetic properties. We also know those countries have used it to get rid of diabetes, which is not currently an accepted statement in the USA. Here's another awesome fact, Gymnema at the time of this writing has no known dangerous side effects (you could have an allergy to it as many of us do). It can also lower your cholesterol.

If used properly, I feel gymnema does have properties where you could supplement your normal diabetic health routine with it. I personally would say go for it however, I cannot highly enough suggest and (if you don't mind) dictate that you talk to your doctor about implementing gymnema before you start using it. From the people I have spoken with, it is extremely rare, as I do not remember hearing one, a doctor will say no! Gymnema anyone? Don't you think it's about time to get on the right diabetic diet side with a little help from gymnema?

Gymnema Will Make You Eat Less Sugar and Lose Weight!
Is that True About Gymnema? Read on!

Can Gymnema prevent sugar cravings? I heard some truth to that and decided to research the topic a bit and I was pretty excited as I'd be learning something new! I am not new at all to fads and health trends that have little to no backing, gymnema hasn't hit that list yet, however something similar to gymnema – hoodia, partially has. I say partially because the truth was expanded and stretched quite a bit. This is not going to be totally about gymnema being your new sweet tooth killer, however it'll be geared more toward advertisements and their potential effect. I'll couple that with my experiences at Vitamin World and a gym I owned. I'll walk across a line that shouldn't be crossed, however normally is, and what it means to you.

Is This Another Advertising Trick Using Gymnema?

Whenever new research shows a possibility of something that will be marketable, companies large and small run with it. Look at hoodia, a plant native to Africa, for example. African hunters and warriors ate the plant to ward off hunger which could be attributed to a couple of things. One, they also drank water when they ate (water is sometimes scare, so eating and drinking at the

same time makes a TON of sense!), and also, like gymnema, they did not grind the plant down from what I've read to make a powder and then place that powder into pill form. Is it illegal for a company to lie? Yep! However, it is not illegal, although it is unethical, is often portrayed as fluffery. Can eating hoodia or using pure hoodia extract aid in appetite suppression? It can, and I have seen it happen at specific concentrations and amounts.

Gymnema could be no different than hoodia in the way advertising companies take over the awesome plant. I will tell you this about gymnema – you will not lose 18 pounds over night! However, can sucking on a gymnema tablet ease your sweet tooth? It may sound outlandish however don't discount yet another gymnema power attribute just yet!

My Take on Gymnema Preventing Sugar Cravings

My take on gymnema preventing sweet tooth or sugar cravings? I say buy into the idea, however let's take a peek at tinctures as well as pills. Talk to your doctor!

Health Benefits From Cinnamon

When I hear cinnamon mentioned a few things come to my mind. It is a tasty treat for breakfast or dessert, it smells very good, and it is in any food store I can think of. If you want a shocker, there are new studies pointing to numerous health benefits from cinnamon on top of its palate pleasing goodness!

Before we talk about some of the numerous health benefits from cinnamon, do you have any idea where it comes from? Cinnamon does naturally come in it's quill form believe it or not. Cinnamon is actually the bark of a specific type of tree, the cinnamon tree (surprise) which is an evergreen type of tree. There is no such thing as plain old cinnamon, in fact there are numerous types of cinnamon! The various forms of cinnamon come from many different parts of Asia.

Most of the world's cinnamon, estimates have the number around 90%, come from Sri Lanka and Southern India while other area's ranging from Madagascar to Vietnam and China produce the remaining 10%. Cassia is one of the types of cinnamon and is the most common form of cinnamon in the United States. Cassia is also known as "Chinese Cinnamon" while "True Cinnamon" is grown in Sri Lanka. Sri Lankan cinnamon has a much more delicate and "high end" taste than what we have grown use to in America.

Not to be outdone, cassia- although not as aromatic – has been used in China for thousands of years for its medicinal properties. Along with the different types of cinnamon, it also comes in a variety of forms. Aside from the common baking powder, you can

take the cinnamon quills or sticks – however if grating bark bothers you creating a liquid from cinnamon is also very easy. You can simply take the quills as they are and place them into a liquid and allow their properties to become infused in what you place them in (for example tea's or milk). Lately there have been numerous types of liquid form cinnamon being produced as well as pill form at any reputable nutritional supplement store.

Now we go onto some of the health benefits from cinnamon. Let's start with digging into your knowledge about this sweet treat. Do you know how potent nutritionally a teaspoon of cinnamon can be? It has vitamins K and C as well as a hefty dose of various minerals. Some of the minerals in that small teaspoon we're talking about will give you 28 milligrams of calcium, just about a gram of iron, as well as some manganese! On top of all of those nutrients, you will also get a useable, non-fibrous, gram of carbs.

I personally started taking this spice for a painful digestive issue I commonly have had since a child, one that can actually affect others as well. Anti-gas is a medicinal health benefit of cinnamon, and I have had my share of pain full (in a physical pain as well as aroma pain sense). I have also found that cinnamon helps me personally with upset stomachs I normally get due to an acid reflux issue. Other digestive health benefits of cinnamon are its ability to combat diarrhea, bloating, indigestion, and some feel nausea.

The gastro-intestinal side of cinnamon isn't the only potent activity packed in here. Cinnamon has started to become very popular in the scientific and medical communities as new health benefits are becoming known. Cinnamon recently has been found to also possess anti-inflammatory effects in a decent amount of various studies. This could be why my mother has less

arthritis pain when she sips cinnamon sticks in her tea to combat the mentioned indigestion.

Diabetic? Here's Why You'll Want Some Cinnamon!

People who have cholesterol or blood glucose problems should be intrigued to find that the mentioned health issues is where the health benefits from cinnamon appear to have the strongest effect!

One such health benefit of cinnamon that medical professionals are looking into is its potentially large effect on insulin resistance as well improving Type 2 diabetes! There have been numerous positive studies on how cinnamon can also improve blood glucose control as well as insulin sensitivity. It only took a half of a teaspoon of cinnamon for these results to begin showing.

If you can manage to improve your insulin resistance, you may not only reduce your dependence on medicine however, you could also lose weight and reduce your risk of heart disease. The studies I am referring to are in the preliminary stages and thus the results are inconclusive and some of the results were mixed. Regardless, a strong portion of the research in these studies is pointing to the health benefits of cinnamon being very beneficial. Aside from improving blood sugar, cinnamon also showed the potential to lower numerous heart disease risks. Some of the risk factors that were noticed was a drop in blood pressure, triglycerides, as well as bad (LDL) cholesterol.

Although cinnamon is relatively harmless, it does possess some anti-clotting properties. People who are taking blood thinners, or aspirin to thin their blood, could in turn encounter some complications with high doses. Another group who should avoid high doses are pregnant women who may encounter stimulation

of the uterus, which could cause some birth or pregnancy complications.

Although preliminary studies on the health benefits from cinnamon are semi-inconclusive and showed mixed results in some cases, the results should not be looked down upon. In fact, this herb has been sought after and highly valued since the days of Moses.

The Diabetic Diet and A1C levels?

What are A1C levels anyway before we think about how the diabetic diet affects them? Your A1C levels are actually a measurement of your average blood sugar levels over the course of 2-3 months. The test is a blood test which is done in your endocrinologist's office. The information given is important, because your endo. needs to know how your levels are normally, especially if you are just starting a diabetic diet.

Finger pricking (I know, it is such a fun activity!) which is done a few times a day is still needed, however the levels fluctuate. Imagine a baseball game, a player can go 4/5 and have a .800 batting average during a game, however through the entire season he could be hitting just .198. Which number is more descriptive of his abilities? The larger picture. That analogy relates to finger pricking and A1C levels and your doctor needs the "big picture" on top of how you hit during the game!

How can the diabetic diet help you? Well, for one you are now on a more healthy diet, as the diabetic diet is more rigid and nutritious. Many of the beans, for example, you could have as part of your plate (the smaller one quarter) will provide additional protein to the other quarter which is strictly protein! The larger portion of your plate will have tons of healthy carbs and fiber that will clean you out on top of providing health benefits! In combination with your medical regime, the diabetic diet could slowly lower your A1C levels.

After being on the diabetic diet, it may make a lot less sense toward why your doctor needs to know your A1C levels at face

value. In all actuality it is pretty imperative. Why? Because your insulin and other medicines will probably have to be adjusted (I've seen numerous times where they were LOWERED!) which is a common, positive side effect of the diabetic diet. Hopefully you can see why this is important, and the fact that the diabetic diet does play a huge role! Another thing your doctor should know is what you normally consume on your diabetic diet!

How can Processed Food Alter the Diabetic Diet?

The diabetic diet has no room for processed food in it, especially since we are creatures of habit. The diabetic diet is not tough to follow, however being creatures of habit the diabetic diet could easily follow the "If You Give a Mouse a Cookie" children's story. I saw a commercial recently where a woman was teasing her spouse I believe to come up with a reason why high fructose corn syrup was bad.

Why Make the Diabetic Diet Tough?

As a diabetic, you know that being on any kind of diet is tough. The diabetic diet is actually easy to follow if you understand some super simple guidelines! One of the more important objectives for you is trying to stay away from processed foods. The commercial I mentioned earlier that I had seen should be considered misleading. High fructose corn syrup is not good for you!

Actually just about any processed food is very bad for you! Why? The answer is simple, when food is processed it changes the food chemical and nutritional makeup and is no longer something your body is accustom to. Look at flour for example, we all know whole grain unbleached flour is not that horrible for us. Why would white flour than be a problem to include in your new diabetic diet? It has been bleached, the goodness that was there has been altered, changed, and broken down. This is a reason why white flour and white sugar can cause your blood sugar to spike a bit. The reason it spikes is that the now super small

processed particles and molecules can be sucked right into your bloodstream.

Will you be paying slightly more for your healthier food? Quite possibly, and if it is tough financially I would really chat with your doctor about Gymnema! The diabetic diet, again, is super easy to follow. Go through your cabinets and read your labels. A very easy rule of thumb I was taught when studying the diabetic diet was that if I could not pronounce it, my body couldn't use it! Again, do not forget you are embarking on the diabetic diet to change your life, make it easy and let the diabetic diet work for you!

Glycine Propionyl L-Carnitine:
Part Amino Acid Part Fat Eater!

Can glycine propionyl l-carnitine be a safe supplement to add to your supplement mix? The diabetic diet can be enhanced tremendously in combination with exercising regularly. When we exercise, we get sore sometimes and some get so sore they are on the "bench" for a week or longer! Let's take a look at how the main ingredients in glycine propionyl l-carnitine can help you and decide if this is something worth discussing with your doctor!

Let us first look at the "bonded" items that make this supplement. What is glycine and what does it do? Aside from being the first word in glycine propionyl l-carnitine, glycine is an amino acid. Don't assume because it is an amino acid you need to begin supplementing it as our bodies normally make sufficient levels on their own.

Another reason you may not need to supplement with glycine is that it is found in the protein of all living, high protein sources. Glycine is the simplest of all amino acids, however don't discount its abilities just yet! It plays a role in things from helping with bile creation to being thought to have an active role in memory! Is Glycine Propionyl L-Carnitine looking better yet?

Glycine propionyl l-carnitine also contains one of my "favorite" supplements, L_Carnitine, which is the last word of glycine propionyl l-carnitine. I have been a huge fan of L-Carnitine for quite some time for its role in helping our mitochondria turn

long chain fats into energy! You could say that L-Carnitine is actually a fat eater! Glycine propionyl l-carnitine has been known to reduce the effects of angina as well as help promote anti aging properties!

Why Use Glycine Propionyl L-Carnitine

So why would someone want to use glycine propionyl l-carnitine or supplement with it? As I had previously mentioned it is pretty nice in reducing post workout soreness. It also helps in the production of creatine which is widely known as being one of the top workout supplements! Actually, glycine propionyl l-carnitine has also been preached about in a study in reducing LAC (blood lactate levels) by over 16%. If you are prediabetic, glycine propionyl l-carnitine has also been known to ward off type 2 diabetes as well as improve heart health.

So in the end, is Glycine Propionyl L-Carnitine something you should talk about with your doctor? I say you should absolutely consider it! Seeing Glycine Propionyl L-Carnitine is diabetic safe I'd highly suggest asking your endocrinologist about how Glycine Propionyl L-Carnitine could affect you!

Diabetic Diet Resources During the Summertime

In New England, we do not always have the hottest temperatures, however these diabetic diet resources can help you stay cool! We all know the summer is fun, in Massachusetts that "fun" can come with a hefty price and you can be in trouble if you aren't using certain seasonal diabetic diet resources. In fact, recently my ex-girlfriend and I took our son for a 2.5ish mile walk around our block. We brought waters and little man had a sippy cup. Around the final 3/4's of our walk, my darling ex-girl started acting funny and started going to town with food from her bag of snacks. She looked completely lost, she was sweating more than me (I am a sweater), and she started really slowing down. Her blood sugar was plummeting! Why though? She cooked at the normal times, it wasn't a long walk by any means we do it regularly, so what happened? She cooked and ate hot foods! Granted she went with foods in her diabetic diet resources, but she increased her body temperature. How can we use the diabetic diet resources we have to prevent summertime blues?

Is water in your diabetic diet resources?

During the summer time, we obviously need to stay cool and drink plenty of water which is one of the best and most pure diabetic diet resources you can have in your arsenal!. Water does do a good job cooling us off, however we can counteract that and make our body work harder by eating hot food. Our body then

has to work harder to cool us down, and when it's working it uses energy. So what do we do? We eat some raw foods from our diabetic diet resources! Raw foods in our diabetic diet resources? Yep! And it'll taste good too like veggies and hummus.

Smart Water can be added to your diabetic diet resources has added electrolytes and I feel a difference when I use that instead of regular h2o. One thing you have to watch is your mineral intake as SmartWater has added minerals, which for most should not be an issue, especially on the diabetic diet resources food list! Another thing you can do is inspect the diabetic diet resources for cool snack ideas. A favorite of mine are roasted chick peas.

On a cool night use this tastebud treasure for a snack full of protein! What I do is I take 3 cans of chickpeas, remove the loose skin (not sure of the proper name), throw some olive oil over them after washing (enough to coat the chickpeas), and add cajun seasoning, wasabi, and sea salt. I let them sit for a few hours so the pea's absorb the oil and seasoning. Let them dry out for about an hour and throw them in the oven at 350 degrees for about an hour. I move them around every 15 minutes to even out the cooking.

Salads can be fun as well! In the food listing inside Escape Diabetes you can literally make about 100 different types of (edible and tasty!) salads. Actually, Escape Diabetes is one of the best diabetic diet resources I have ever come across. I actually would put it up there along the ranks of "The Maker's Diet" by Jordan Rubin. The food listing, aside from the importance of numerous factors, is very well laid out and breaks food down by important factors. Nothing is wrong with revising your diabetic diet resources. In fact, you can base meals around seasonal diabetic diet resources meal ideas!

Water Is Your New Diabetic Diet Resources Best Friend!

There could be hundreds of diabetic diet resources, only one of those diabetic diet resources however fits the following riddle! What one of the numerous diabetic diet resources fit the following riddle? It makes up most of your body and most of the earth? If you guessed water you are on point! I am not talking about mineral enhanced water, or flavored water. I am talking about the water that flows from mountain springs. The water in the ocean. The plain water we get from our faucet to clean things!

Diabetic Diet Resources are powerful, but WATER Made it?

Why on earth would something as subtle as water be considered a diabetic diet resources powerhouse? It's cleaning properties are first on my list and is one of the few diabetic diet resources around that can claim to clean you! If you are wondering, I am talking about the internal cleansing ability it has over the external, there are diabetic diet resources that are external in use only, not this diabetic diet resource though. I actually found this out through my own observation.

I use to play with something recreationally and needed a job, this is before I was as into diabetic diet resources as I am now. I got a phone call inviting me to an interview, however I was told a cup and a specimen from me would be needed to finalize the hiring process. I freaked out and began drinking water. I am not talking about a couple of cups. I went to Hess and purchased 10 gallons of water! The more I went to the bathroom, the more something

stuck out. My urine was going from a dark yellow color to a clear and transparent color. That brought out the geek in me. That also brought water onto the "major importance" side of my diabetic diet resources list.

During my period of high stress, drinking that water was apparently cleaning my body from the inside out! The research I started doing led me to realize I would not have to buy a super expensive "cleansing drink". I also read that adding some drops of lemon water would cleanse my body a bit more! It actually turns out that water turned into one of my favorite diabetic diet resources! It's God's cleaning agent given to us. I would say that this diabetic diet resources top ranker is free, however now there are aisles full of water at grocery stores, go figure. Make sure you add water to your list of diabetic diet resources!

WHY is Alkaline Water Important?

I figure I'd be doing you an injustice if I did not start off with why it's important to drink alkaline water. I will be talking about pH drops to alkalize your water, but let's grab a quick (I'll try and keep this to only half the amount of the King James Bible – kidding, shooting for a half page at the most! Did you realize this is adding to your reading? Done! Promise, just having a sense of humor moment). Alkaline water is important, and that has some pretty good scientific backing – no-debunking. I'll walk you through the process, but watch the video on alkaline water.

What happens when you drop a simple little tooth into soda? At first, absolutely nothing. What happens after a week, or maybe 2 months? Let's go with two months. Remember, we're not talking alkaline water yet, simple soda. Any regular pop. The good fizzy stuff that goes down oh so smooth? Why would you want to drink alkaline water anyway when a cold refreshing soda does the trick? Well, actually there's an issue. Over time and not checking on it, it appears the tooth fairy stole it! If you believe it was that and that it had nothing to do with a lack of alkaline and extreme amounts of acid, give me your address and tell me when you put the $500 "tooth fairy fee" under your pillow. No, what actually happened is the enamel around your tooth is done, kaput, no longer in existence. Over time, a lack of alkaline water and a huge amount of acid will do that. Imagine drinking battery acid, maybe some form of a weaker semi-ingestible acid. The same could happen to your body all over inside. It is acid!

Why Do We Need to Increase Our Alkaline Water Intake?

Our bodies are very acidic, especially if you stay away from alkaline water and other diabetic diet resources! Alkaline water is something you should try and consume every morning, maybe a couple times a day. You can buy alkalizers all over the place, however you should make it some form of a goal (preferably short-term) to increase your body's pH and maybe take a few swigs of alkaline water instead of acidic soda. It's upto you, of course, however just remember the "tooth" example (and you really don't have to drop your address, if you want to mail me the $500, well I was joking about that also). In closing, alkaline water needs to be increased dramatically. I am not talking about (although there's nothing wrong with it) Smart Water, I am talking alkaline water. How do we alkalize water? Stay tuned =-) I will teach you how to make your own alkaline water.

Alkaline Water : Do It Yourself Style!

Welcome back diabetic diet resource fans and as promised, this section is going to cover alkaline water the do it yourself way! It will take some getting used to, maybe a trial and error however, what do you have to lose? You can certainly buy into Kagen (I believe it's the name of the company) or buy a massive apparatus that you either put on your home's system or faucet for your alkaline water, but why? Last I checked consumer spending was taking a nose dive and hundreds of thousands were becoming more frugal (I've been there for a while!). Let's drink alkaline water. Without paying the alkaline water price tag.

Ready for some Alkaline Water Fun?

I've been drinking alkaline water for a while now, and I have to tell you I feel very, very different when the water I down isn't alkaline! Want to scare yourself? Go buy a couple test strips and take some "purified" bottled water. It should be alkaline water because it's processed and the nasty stuff is removed, right? Did you do the test yet? Okay, say the answer with me now..WRONG. The tests I've done myself show very little to no difference in the alkalinity of different bottled water to traditional tap water. We know alkalinity is important and waters a miracle, so how do we get alkaline water with drops? Go to the next paragraph and you will see how I make it every single day!

Without Further Adieu, How to Make Your Own Alkaline Water

To create alkaline water, and start reversing the acidic problem going on inside you, buy a large lemon. A LEMON? Yes, grab a lemon and a sterilized knife (has little to do with alkalinity, I am use to working in a Kosher approved plant years ago). Cut the lemon into quarters. Take a 16 ounce glass of room temperature water (I'm always thirsty for some reason so the 8 ounce glass does not suit me well) and squeeze the daylights (or juice, just a bit of humor) out of one of your quarters into the water. Stir it with the knife (or spoon, maybe a straw) and you now have alkaline water!

Fast Diabetic Diet Resources

Living in New England is amazing, especially with our natural abundance of diabetic diet resources. The autumn season here is especially phenomenal with breathtaking harvest season views. I love walking and scoping the colorful foliage. Unfortunately, sometimes a hike can be as dangerous as it is beautiful if you don't have a protein and complex carbohydrate dense snack. What can we use from the list of diabetic diet resources that will not require we bring a fork and knife? How about nice and small diabetic diet resources, diabetic diet resources that you can throw into a brown paper bag! You can go with sunflower seeds, roasted chickpeas, and maybe some dried fruit (organic would be best).

I love Autumn, it is my favorite time of year and one of my favorite diabetic diet resources is about to become very easy to find! Maybe not find, but there will be enough of this one that anyone on some form of diabetes diets can add to their diabetic diet resources and make fast! I lied, they are always around, a tasty diabetic diet resources player, mass produced and sold in supermarkets and convenience stores. During October many even decorate with these guys, can you guess what I'm hinting at? If you guessed pumpkin seeds you are on point! I make these little diabetic diet resources pretty much the same way I make my chick pea "nuts"

Diabetic diet resources should be picked with care, not everything makes the diabetic diet resources list! Soybeans are another tasty treat that easily made the cut. Not a whole bunch of fat, but a ton of protein. Not just any protein, but the heart

healthy type! Soybeans yield a larger serving size than most snack items and they are easy to dry out and are compatible with a ton of different flavorings and seasonings. How does that sound for a different diabetic diet resources change of taste? Speaking of taste, when they are cooking consider some wasabi!

Being allergic to peanuts according to a recent allergy test (I was fatally allergic as a child and assumed that had not changed) I need a diabetic diet resources heavy hitter that packs a protein punch. I started throwing a little more cumin in there, ditched the thyme and added cajun seasoning as well as chile's and let me tell you – I created an A+ chick pea snack!

If you like variety, take each of those diabetic diet resources and mix them together for a spicy and salty trail mix! Don't' forget your alkaline water!

Naturally Lower Blood Sugar Levels With Food?

Watch your blood sugar, check your blood sugar, everyone tells you about blood sugar but what about how to naturally lower blood sugar with food? The first time I heard you could naturally lower blood sugar with food I was sceptical as well. If you think about it, there is a very popular old wives tale that talks about processed foods raising your blood sugar faster (think potato chips).

If the unnatural foods raise your blood sugar levels, would it make sense for good, whole, and beneficial foods to naturally lower your blood sugar levels? I think there is a case to be made in favor of the whole foods actually and that case is its ability to naturally lower blood sugar.

What types of foods would do the trick of being able to naturally lower blood sugar? A good place to start is with the soluble fiber found inside of oatmeal. A serving of oatmeal also comes packed with a healthy amount of carbohydrates. This healthy and traditional breakfast staple is known to not only provide a very slow release of sugar, but can also naturally lower blood sugar or at least provide a stable environment in terms of your blood sugar. Does it seem easy to naturally lower blood sugar yet?

Naturally Lower Blood Sugar With This Afternoon Snack

Another food that is real popular is one that neither I nor my children can eat are peanuts. Peanuts are a good snack, can give

your plate a crunchy and salty kick. Peanuts have been thought to naturally lower blood sugar as well.Another form of peanuts can also naturally lower your blood sugar is peanut butter. Peanut butter not only has the slow released carbohydrates for sustained energy, however also contained in those little nuts is protein. While adding muscle building protein, we are also finding naturally lower blood sugar levels!

Lean meat has been thought to naturally lower blood sugar however I am not entirely sold on that idea. Something inside of that lean meat tells another story on how to naturally lower blood sugar, that hidden gem is chromium. Chromium, an important mineral, has long been known to stabilize blood sugar levels, however during my time working at Vitamin World many customers swore that it naturally lowered blood sugar as well. The thought does has a bunch of scientific evidence supporting that claim as we discovered earlier.

We came up with 3 different foods known to or thought to naturally lower blood sugar levels. Is it the food themselves? Well yes and no, in oatmeal and peanut (and peanut butter) it is the long released or complex carbohydrates. Aside from protein and chromium, lean meat also contains some important amino acids. In closing, while the foods themselves could naturally lower blood sugar levels it is the nutrient density that is far more important.

Diabetic Blunders and Myths To Avoid!

I heard something that peaked my interest recently, and made me want to look into and maybe add another diabetic dieting tips! The thought came from overhearing a conversation at a Stop and Shop supermarket in the organic food section. They were talking about diabetic dieting and made it seem as if nature discriminated against diabetics. That made me really think until they mentioned some common sense. Diabetic dieting tips are very similar to the diet help available to everyone. In all actuality, the ones I looked up were the exact same as basic tips for everyone.

That was fine and dandy but it really got me thinking. It actually got me thinking about not just diabetic dieting tips, but wrong information (talk about a curveball!) It also made me really wonder, not in a discriminating way, that could really affect not only a dieting quest by a diabetic, but their health as well.

Here are some of the "Diabetic Dieting Tip" blunders you should avoid:

Our first diabetic dieting tip is not staying up past bedtime! If you're a diabetic, and I'll go out on a limb and assume you are, you need to rest your body! Actually a recent study showed that individuals who had only 4 hours of sleep over a 5 day period took in an additional 300 plus calories per day! YIKES! Talked about a total a wasted effort. That makes this a diabetic dieting tips don't!

Another tip is that you shouldn't be so stringent and tough on yourself with your diet. Granted you are going to want results, however what happens when you attempt to make a child do something they do not want to do? They rebel, and where do you think they learned that trick? Forcing yourself to adhere to a strict diet cold turkey, could give you adverse effects, the main one being you say "forget it".

Granted you probably don't have your eyes set (and why not?) on getting six pack abs, setting lofty, or overly optimistically set goal, could doom you for failure off the bat. Not reaching your goals is going to depress you, but if you set your dieting and weight loss goals so unreasonably high your easiest milestones could take a lifetime.

There are a few important diabetic dieting tips don'ts for you. Take them to heart, and let yourself enjoy success with dieting. Catch you soon!

Some More Myths for You!

I was talking to my friend Russ recently. We were talking about the typical thing, "James you're doing too much" "why the heck did Huntsman drop out of the race and we went with Romney?!?" and other things. We started talking about diabetic diet resources in general and how I just added a whole bunch of weight management tips to this book. I was curious how I could add to that. He said something totally unrelated to the new 'segment' (which always happens with me, random things spark an idea) and I shouted diet myth! What do you think? Let's get started!

Weight loss, fat burning, weight management, and anything you can think about regarding the topics (even how to gain weight) has some friendly advice you've heard, or someone else heard from someone's uncle and they repeated it. Off the bat, the old wive's tales are not always a bunch of sugary crap – however they could be distorted a la the game of "telephone". Do you remember that game? It actually should be added as a real small sub category to your diabetic diet resources list. I know, I know, hold on a minute though. What happens during 'telephone'? A message starts out as a whisper into one ear, and continues from one mouth to one ear via whisper. Normally at the end, the message can go from "I need some water" to "the Astrodome was flooded by a bunch of giraffe's that couldn't hold it anymore", know what I mean?

Where do Diet Myths Come From?

Diet myths can come in all shapes and sizes, one I actually heard was that it is easier to burn fat during certain stages of the moon (WHAT?!). Diabetic diet resources can come in all shapes and sizes ranging from say blood sugar monitoring to telephone to weight management.

Let me start with the first diet myth. Fruit juices are good for you and you should consume them whenever you get a chance for vitamins and minerals. Is it a diet myth, or is there truth to this one? To an extent both answers are correct actually, depending how you look at them. Fruit and vegetables are high (some are insanely) high in good vitamins, protein, and so on. The problem, if you are like me eating raw vegetables is more of a task than a pleasure. The alternative is to cook them which makes them taste super good, but wastes out a ton of the good stuff God made them come with automatically.

Are Cooked Vegetables Good for You or is That a Diet Myth?

Seeing cooked vegetables lose a lot of their nutritional density (I am NOT saying they are bad for you, they are still an awesome diabetic diet resources top pick), you may think that fruits are a better alternative. Maybe, how is your sugar today would be the first question I ask you though? Good, great consider it. Are you going to bring a corer for an apple or a peeler for other fruits? Where is the lemon (my sons eat straight up lemons, how I don't know but they love them!) or grapefruit rind going to go?

Seeing you probably do not have a portable trash bag with you (unless you're a neat freak or a super parent), I can't see you throwing your rinds and peels on the floor of your car. Plus your hands are going to get all messy and sticky, and during the summer time you'll be basically asking for all kinds of scary flying and stinging insects to hang out on your hands (that would be an instant freak out for me by the way – terrified of bees and their relatives). The diet myth is on its way don't worry, actually the diet myth is making an appearance in the paragraph below!

Starting to Sound Like a Diet Myth to Me!

We don't carry trash cans with us, not too many have sani-wipes in their pockets at all times, there is a law against littering. That means the only alternative we have is fruit juices, and to this I say welcome to the diet myth!

If you visit any grocery store or supermarket you see them all over the place. A while back, I mentioned processed foods so keep that thought in mind. The juices are dressed up and labeled in all sorts of sex appealed ways. "High in Vitamin C", "The Highest Antioxidant Count", "A full serving of vitamin C and B in each serving" are a couple of the highlights I pulled from an ad for Hannaford Brother's.

Although those look like amazing points, and they are as vitamin C and antioxidant properties are crucial in today's world more than ever for your health. Maybe not more than ever, however with our health as a nation there's no debating the urgency to add these to your diets mask other things in a lackluster product. Remember I asked how your sugar was a few paragraphs ago? Look at the back of the bottle. Some fruit juices can contain as much as 52 grams of sugar PER SERVING – not good for those of us into diabetic diet resources.

Fruit juices are also processed, which adds to the diet myth (mainly for us diabetic diet resources fanatics – but it does include everyone period – processing isn't the best form of nutrition for you!). The alternative, do you think there's an alternative?

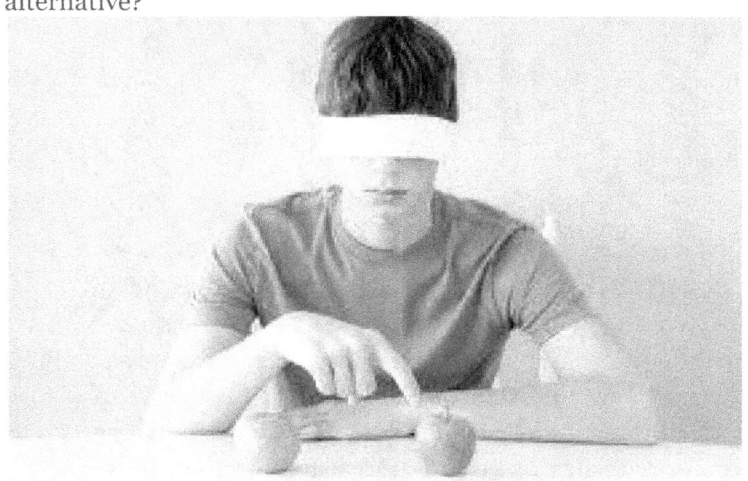

How about fresh juiced – juice? I mean where you take maybe a broccoli stem (a HA!), some kale, maybe a small serving of eggplant, some strawberries and blueberries (for taste of course) and drink that? Right there, I see iron, vitamin C, antioxidants, flavonoids, vitamin K (does your diabetes make it harder for you to clot? Your vitamin K could be helping you as soon as you start sipping!), and tons of other very healthy items. Oh, and good carbs too, we can't forget those. You also have a fruity taste to it!

Am I a professional juicer? No way, that's Barry Bonds' (another baseball reference, God I can't wait for Spring Training) specialty. I read on it here and there, however I throw my trash on my car floor and carry sani-wipes with me. Plus working a few hours a week as a merchandiser (everyone needs to find a way to get out of the house and socialize!) I touch all kinds of germy things at the store.

If you are looking into juicing the right way, you really need to look at this as it could be a solid addition to your diabetic diet resources.

Is There A Diabetic Exercise?

When it comes to diabetic diet resources one of the most important tools you have is your safety, and almost equally important as food is a diabetic exercise! A diabetic exercise? That sounds as to me as it probably does to you, there is no such thing. Maybe taking your insulin and injecting it, however where is the calorie burning there? Maybe if you created a diabetic exercise that used isometric exercise as a basis for injecting? It's a foolish thought as diabetics are no different than you and I aside from, well, diabetes.

As a former personal trainer, I understand how daunting admitting an injury or condition that limits you can be and it should be a very wise consideration to "open yourself up a bit". Do not be upset if you get a smirk when you ask for a diabetic exercise routine, also when you ask for a diabetic exercise routine you may receive a puzzled look – it is natural when talking about diabetic exercise!

Wait, there's no such thing as a diabetic exercise routine?!

Now, is there a such thing as a diabetic exercise you should have in your diabetic diet resources? I am going to go out on a limb and say diabetic exercise is the exact same as any other exercise. The main difference is when a diabetic exercises, blood sugar maintenance and checking need to happen before and mid-workout. Do you know why? Yes! You answered your blood sugar could plummet especially during hard strenuous exercises, right? Well if not that is the answer anyway.

A diabetic exercise routine will contain some red flags for the personal trainer, and if you mention you are afflicted with diabetes and ask for a diabetic exercise routine, many trainers will simply say no. If you still want to label it as a diabetic exercise or diabetic exercise routine, you have to realize you are a potential liability and depending on the trainers insurance you may get shot down upon uttering anything diabetic exercise related.

If you want to imagine there is a diabetic exercise, let's use a timeline to describe it. As part of your diabetic diet resources we have diet and exercise (plus more to come!). If you have just recently began an exercise program, wouldn't it be a wise idea to talk to a personal trainer and learn a few "moves"? Of course it would, being a personal trainer I always asked the detective questions, as everyone already 'knows everything' and I was just there for an opinion (I call it the 7 year old attitude). If they had a heart problem or diabetes I NEEDED to know. Not to custom create an exercise regimen, but to know if I had to watch out for additional warning signs!

Diabetic exercise is a very easy item to get around, and in fact I know many who swear there are various diabetic exercise routines, they always get mad when I giggle at them. Diabetic exercise is no different than you and me exercising. Although I was pre-diabetic I never looked into a diabetic exercise (probably because I didn't exercise so why would I bother with a diabetic exercise?).

Although there is no diabetic exercise routine, nor is there any form of diabetic exercise protocol, is that to say a diabetic cannot achieve say six pack abs? Absolutely not! You just have to be more cautious and if you take on a trainer you need to let them know you are diabetic, but leave out the diabetic exercise talk!

An Important Task – Weight Management

Weight management is an, unfortunately, very minimally discussed topic. If you are one of the millions who pledge to lose weight and have succeeded, congratulations! However, a diet is not made to last forever, unless it is a diabetes diets idea, and after the diet comes weight management to ensure the pounds you lost remain found by someone aside from you.

From my experience as a personal trainer, especially for high risk diabetic clients, there are going to be three steps you want to ensure you follow. Following these steps after one of the diabetes diets out there should dramatically increase your chances of weight management success! Those three steps for weight management success are: preparation, focus, and belief.

Preparing for Weight Management Success

Preparing for weight management is actually extremely easy, so much so it is often assumed (by you) that you do not need to write it down. Prepare yourself and you will do fine! You should weigh yourself everyday after your diet and find your new normal weight! Keep track of your numbers and if you end up slipping you will catch it and get back on track!

Prepare your meals ahead of time can make dinner an easier task and also make healthy eating an easy new, and very good, habit. You'll also have the list in front of you which is needed (maybe) for your shopping list! Go with the standard diabetic diet resources plan with the 1/4, 1/4, and 1/2 portions.

The Shopping List and Weight Management – Accelerate Your Weight Management Success!

A shopping list being created ahead of time is a good starting point. What's good for you that you do not have? You would put that on your list. This is pretty important if you have a junk food habit. You can also, seeing you are planning your "shopping trip attack", follow the money saving diabetic diet resources new addition – coupons! I cannot tell you how many times I went shopping without a list and had to go back for the things I really went there for. Normally I get nothing I knew I needed and get into a bad mood (I hate wasting time). Make your life easier and just write your list (and remember to bring it!).

Weight management starts with what you eat!

A big weight management practice is exercise, however, after you burn all that belly fat you are probably going to assume your work is done. That is a huge mistake, you need to plan for consistency or you will end up back on a diet when there is no reason for it.

You want to remain vigilant when it comes to planning your gym trips. I have found that this is the area that starts getting neglected most often after a diet. Plan on getting to the gym about 20 times monthly and you may surprise yourself by following your plan! Does planning seem a bit easier now?

Focus on This Weight Management Tip For Success!

Here is another tip for you on weight management! If your memory serves you correctly, you should recall that I mentioned there are three different principles for weight management success. In the previous tip I touched on the preparation aspect. That included planning ahead and coming up with lists and such. That part is important for this aspect, the weight management principal on focus.

Weight Management Demands Focus!

Although focus is imperative for weight management to work for you, you really need to make a conscious effort to plan ahead of time. If you are ready for something, say a test, you can sit down and get moving on the questions, right? Preparation was the easier tip, I am not saying that focus isn't entirely easy – it is once you get moving with it, however it will be tougher for you to stay focused and on track if you don't have the supplies you need on hand.

A very good question you may have is how focus works into your weight management goals. The easiest way I can answer that is I am going to assume you have had tough days before. A tough day can, if you are not focused, turn into a tough week very easily. As a diabetic, or have diabetic concerns, you can appreciate that every once in awhile your blood sugar doesn't do what you want.

You may also be upset that you didn't prepare yourself for this week properly. A main goal of the focus portion for weight management is to realize the outcome is your least concern. You are learning what and how to prepare and focus. Focusing on the process will make the outcome you desire far more easy to reach.

Can Alkaline Water Help You Reach Your Weight Management Goals?

One item you want to focus on for weight management is your alkaline water consumption. Granted you could drink regular filtered tap water, however diabetes is something I'd rather "go the extra mile" for, do you agree? Alkaline water intake has shown to not improve only your health, however your vitality as well as other aspects of your daily life.

Another word for focus is consistency, and that new term works right into following a weight management approach. One item you want to be consistent with is your exercise patterns. Focus on not allowing the thought "I will just go tomorrow" to become a common excuse for you to skip a workout. If you missed one planned trip focus on telling yourself you will not miss the next one. Those little cues can act as reaffirmation and increase your chances of doing so!

Weight Management Is Very Demanding, Especially With Consistency!

Another weight management aspect that you really must focus on is eating the same amount of meals at the same time. Not only will this work in your favor in regards to stabilizing your blood sugar, you will find yourself being regularly full. Another aspect of your personal health this will work for is keeping your metabolism working at a regular and consistent pace.

A main diabetic diet resources principal is that you want to have the "diabetic diet" plate breakdown. That is one quarter of your plate is lean meat, another quarter is starchy food, while the last half portion is non-starchy carbohydrates. This is another aspect you really need to focus on as you will be giving your body food it can turn into energy, and not relying on protein as an energy source. That's a weight management tip you should be using already!

Those are the weight management tips for the focus portion. There are not any others I can place in the level of importance that these get. One thing I will repeat is that you can not stress over having a bad day. Doing so will decrease your focus while increasing your risk of failure.

Weight Management – You have to Believe In It!

In the previous weight management tips we touched on what weight management was, why you should consider it, focus, and preparation. This final tip will talk about the third weight management task and could hold the cliche "save the best for last" true. Belief in yourself and your abilities is critical for not only regarding weight management but rather any aspect of your life. Actually if you consider it all three of the weight management principles we went over so far are items that will give you not only success with your diabetes, but improve you as a person also.I have always said confidence, but not arrogance, is always a winning pick in life.

Weight Management Will Be Tough, I believe In You!

At times, you are going to find the going tough. Weight management, understandably, is going to be considered being placed on your 'back burner'. We all have tough times, and we all have constraints where unnecessary tasks are put on hold. When it comes to your health, it may seem that a temporary pause for something that is only supplemental. If you are taking bilberry for your eyes and your life is really so hectic you can't take a single pill that day, so be it. Are thing like that really that time consuming though, or are you simply easily frustrated?It is times like these you need to stop for a moment and think like a winner.

Actually, having a positive thought processes and trying to maintain that will make weight management all the more bearable for you. I have already mentioned at times it is going to not only be tough, but potentially daunting. It may even be fair to assume weight management is tough when you first go into it. It should also be known that weight management is a lifestyle change, and what lifestyle change has ever been easy?

Thinking positively will allow you to consider how many have done it before you and come to the realization that if they can achieve weight management, why can't you? That concept isn't only tied down to weight management, anything you can envisioned has had people either succeed or fail at it, it is up to you to decide how your experience will go.

Dr. Peale Helped Me With Weight Management!

Dr. Norman Vincent Peale was a world class author and mentor in the topic of positive thoughts and its rewards. In fact, one of Dr. Peale's best pieces was the "Power of Positive Thinking". That is probably one of the single best written books as far as implementable insight into transforming your life.

Positive thinking, occasionally, can only go so far though and you will literally have to depend on your memory to continue down the road with weight management. I am not saying you will develop Alzheimer's as a result of merely having diabetes, however you will probably find yourself saying "why should I even bother?" Weight management is not a process where you will see instant results, so you can't really be blamed for considering that once in awhile. In times like these you need your memory to reflect on the accomplishments you've had or milestones you've reached.

In The End, You Can Achieve Weight Management Success, If You Let Yourself!

It's easy to understand why you may feel like throwing in the towel, however with this information at your disposal, it's even easier to understand why you are expecting success with weight management. Accepting that weight management is a process, and really being proud of yourself for reaching those tough to hit milestones will really help you stay the course and enjoy weight management success!

You Made It This Far!

So what do you think, can you naturally improve diabetes? Legally in the USA you can't say yes, even doctors will not give you a straight yes, but they won't say no either. We've covered a type - juvenile - that's not curable at all. But can you reduce the symptoms? Absolutely, if you know what you're doing!

We've covered tips, how to avoid getting laughed at, things you can supplement with your doctor's approval. We've looked at some evidence, and some theory. We covered a LOT in this short book.

I'd like it if you would give me a review, it'll help me spread the word and help other's learn options they may be able to use themselves!

Aside from a review, if you liked or at least found this book interesting would you be kind enough to tell 5 friends or family members about it?

Here are a few additional resources you should consider, especially since now you know there's no specific "diabetic exercise"!